I0720845

LOAN GORDON

Quick Guide to Essential Oils

How skin and tummy issues led me to the top 10 essential oils

Copyright © 2023 by Loan Gordon

All rights reserved. No part of this publication may be reproduced, stored or transmitted in any form or by any means, electronic, mechanical, photocopying, recording, scanning, or otherwise without written permission from the publisher. It is illegal to copy this book, post it to a website, or distribute it by any other means without permission.

Loan Gordon asserts the moral right to be identified as the author of this work.

Loan Gordon has no responsibility for the persistence or accuracy of URLs for external or third-party Internet Websites referred to in this publication and does not guarantee that any content on such Websites is, or will remain, accurate or appropriate.

Designations used by companies to distinguish their products are often claimed as trademarks. All brand names and product names used in this book and on its cover are trade names, service marks, trademarks and registered trademarks of their respective owners. The publishers and the book are not associated with any product or vendor mentioned in this book. None of the companies referenced within the book have endorsed the book.

First edition

This book was professionally typeset on Reedsy.
Find out more at reedsy.com

Contents

Preface

My journey with essential oils started out of a longtime struggle with persistent and unexplainable skins rashes and tummy turmoil. It didn't help that I am gluten intolerant, lactose intolerant, and allergic to nuts (except almonds...phew!). I wasn't about to let these health issues interfere with living and enjoying life.

Determined to overcome my annoying skin, hair, and stomach pains, I put my love for reading and research to work on a journey to self-diagnosis and awareness—and voilà! I found the path to essential oil enlightenment and more.

At first, my trials and tribulations in essential oils were natural remedies to symptoms of skin itchiness and redness, and stomach aches and bloating. Then, it blossomed into an eagerness to learn more about natural health, clean beauty, and overall, a healthier way of living in terms of what I put in, on, and around my body.

My journey to healthier living has been 20 years in the making. Today, I am intentional about what I put into my body and the products I use, opting for more natural, chemical-free, and less-processed choices when possible. It's not 100%, and I'm not fanatical about it, but I will try my best. Because of these changes, and the essential oil products I have developed and use daily, I feel better, and I am healthier.

I hope this quick guide gives you just that—a quick introduction to the vast field of essential oils and aromatherapy. It is by no means an extensive book. As an essential oil beginner, it's a starting point for you to embark upon your own personal journey of research and exploration into the wonderful world of essential oils.

Many thanks for reading my book, and have a wonderful essential oil journey.

1

Introduction

Welcome to the "Quick Guide to Essential Oils," a primer for kickstarting your exploration into the fascinating world of essential oils.

This guide introduces you to the essence of these natural wonders— highly concentrated plant extracts renowned for their unique scents and myriad benefits. Whether you are a novice intrigued by the allure of natural fragrances or a seasoned enthusiast seeking deeper knowledge, this guide offers a clear, concise overview of the top 10 essential oils and their uses.

As we embark on this aromatic journey, we will uncover the extraction methods that capture the pure essence of plants, the diverse properties and compositions of these oils, and their practical applications across various domains. From the soothing ambiance of aromatherapy and the therapeutic touch in topical applications to the natural efficiency in household products and the gentle healing in natural remedies, essential oils offer a harmonious blend of nature's best for your health, home, and heart.

Join me in navigating this fragrant world, understanding the safety considerations and quality aspects that ensure an enriching experience with these potent extracts. Prepare to immerse yourself in the enchanting world of essential oils, a journey that promises to be as enlightening as it is fragrant.

2

Understanding Essential Oils

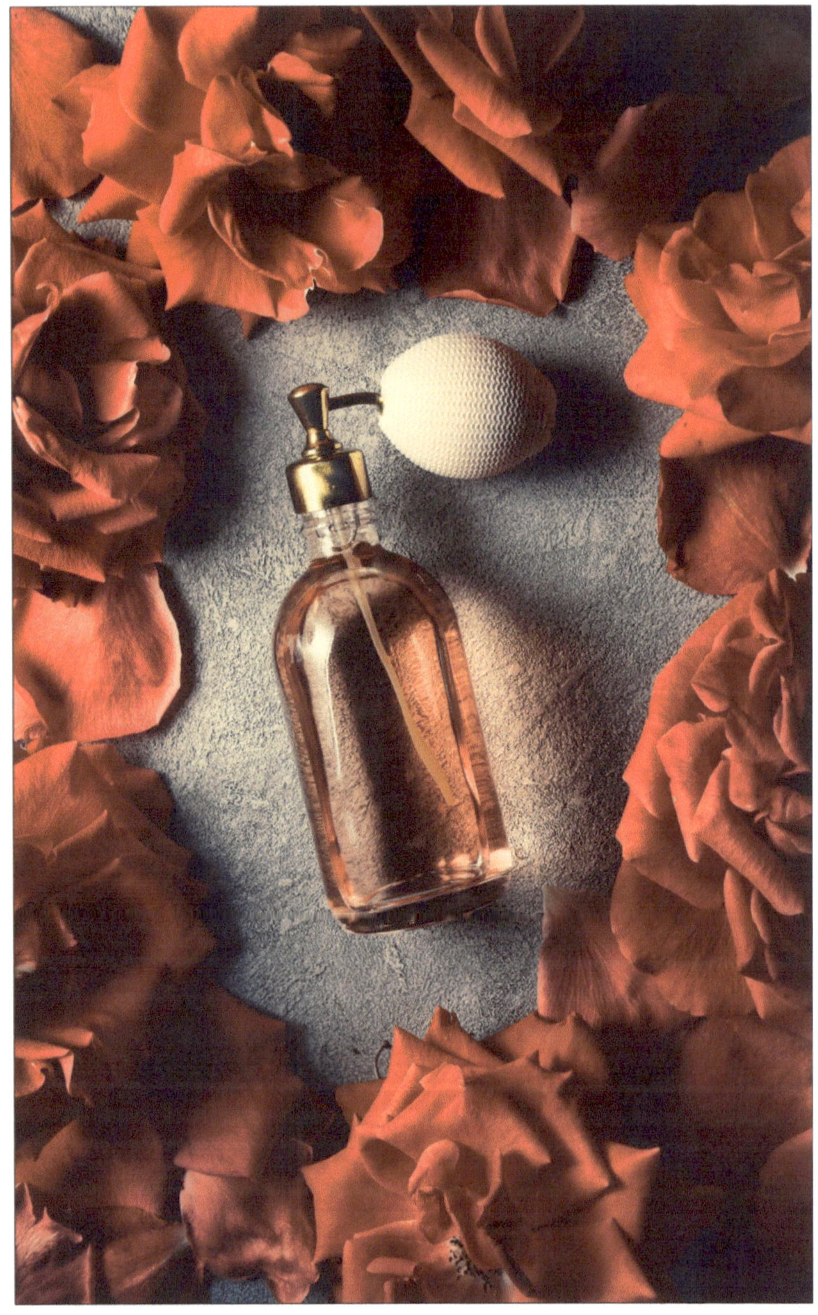

Essential oils are highly concentrated natural oils extracted from plants. They are known for their distinctive scents and are often used in aromatherapy, cosmetics, alternative medicine, household products, and personal care.

Extraction Methods

Essential oils are natural substances extracted from various parts of plants, including leaves, flowers, bark, roots, and peels. The process of extracting these oils is critical in preserving their aromatic and therapeutic properties.

The most prevalent method is steam distillation, where steam passes through the plant material, vaporizing the volatile compounds. These vapors are then cooled and condensed back into a liquid form, capturing the essence of the plant. Cold pressing, another extraction technique, is primarily used for citrus oils. In this method, the plant material is mechanically pressed to release the oils without using heat, ensuring the preservation of delicate compounds. Solvent extraction, on the other hand, is reserved for extremely heat-sensitive materials such as jasmine or rose. This method involves using solvents to gently extract the aromatic compounds.

Each of these extraction methods plays a crucial role in maintaining the integrity, purity, and unique characteristics of essential oils.

Properties and Composition

Essential oils are distinguished by their highly concentrated nature, making them far more potent than the plants from which they are derived. This potency is a result of their unique composition, as each oil contains a complex blend of natural compounds. These compounds are responsible for the distinctive aromas and therapeutic properties of the oils, varying significantly from one oil to another.

Another key characteristic of essential oils is their volatility. They are prone to rapid evaporation at room temperature, a trait that allows them to release their robust and often therapeutic aromas into the air. This volatility is not only central to their use in aromatherapy but also contributes to their effectiveness in various applications, from natural remedies to enhancing the ambiance of a space.

The combination of high concentration, unique composition, and volatility makes essential oils a fascinating and versatile component in both traditional and modern practices.

3

Essential Oil Uses

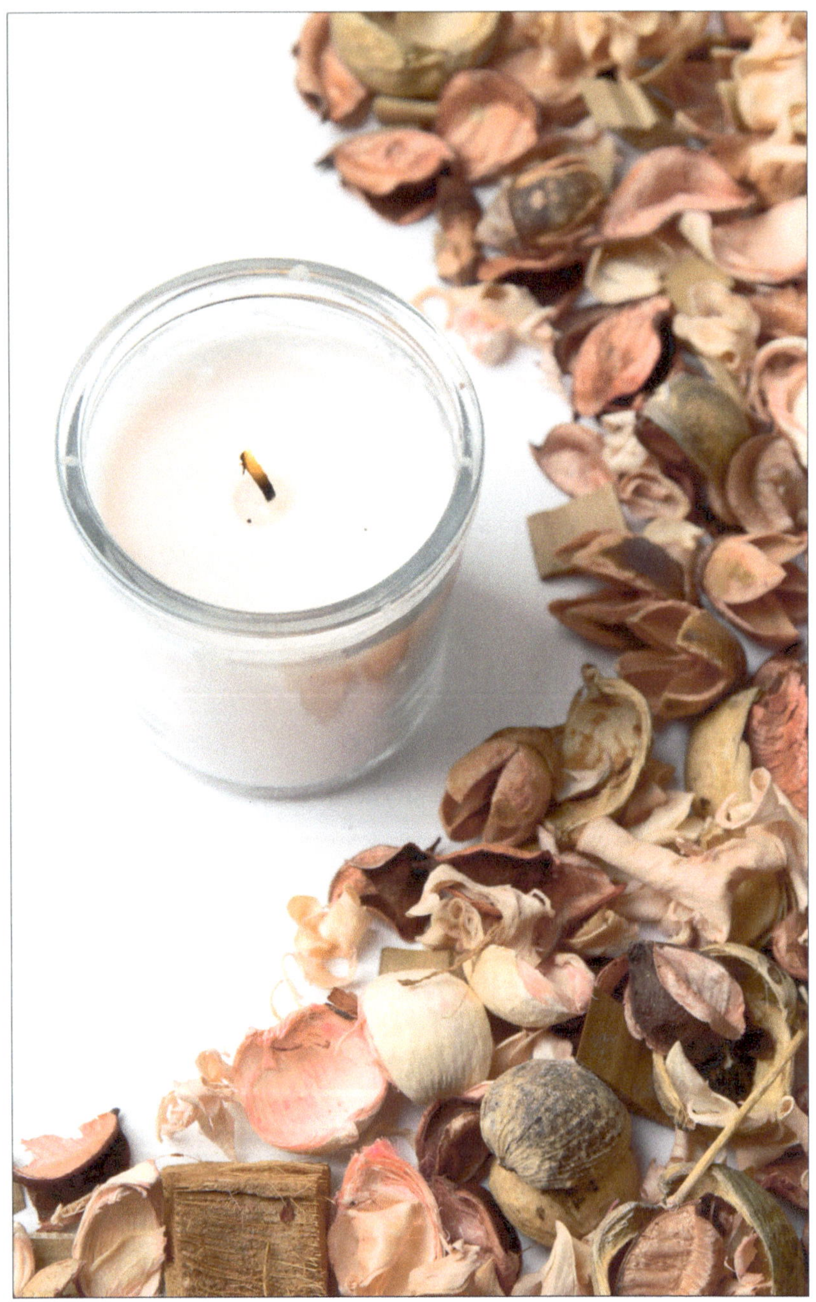

Essential oils, with their diverse and potent properties, find their use in a variety of domains, ranging from wellness practices to household applications.

Aromatherapy

Aromatherapy with essential oils is a holistic practice that harnesses the aromatic compounds of plants for therapeutic benefit. In this practice, essential oils are inhaled, typically using diffusers, which disperse the oil's particles into the air. The inhalation of these aromatic molecules is believed to stimulate the olfactory system—the part of the brain connected to smell. As the aroma molecules reach the brain, they can affect the limbic system, which plays a role in emotions, behaviors, sense of smell, and long-term memory. This is why aromatherapy is often used for stress relief, mood enhancement, and even to improve cognitive functions like focus and memory.

Popular oils for aromatherapy include lavender, known for its calming effects, peppermint for its invigorating properties, and eucalyptus for its refreshing and decongestant qualities. Aromatherapy can be practiced in various settings, from personal spaces like homes to professional environments like spas, offering a natural and non-invasive method to enhance physical and emotional well-being.

Topical Applications

The use of essential oils in topical applications, particularly in massage and skincare, is a testament to their versatility and therapeutic benefits. When applied to the skin, these oils can provide various benefits, such as soothing muscle tension, enhancing skin health, and promoting relaxation. However, due to their high concentration, essential oils are typically diluted with a carrier oil, like sweet almond, jojoba, or coconut oil, to prevent skin irritation and enhance absorption. This dilution makes the application safer and facilitates a smoother massage experience, allowing the oil to glide easily over the skin.

In skincare, essential oils are used for their specific properties—tea tree oil for its antimicrobial qualities, Frankincense for anti-aging, or lavender for its calming and soothing effects. The application of these oils can be tailored to individual skin types and concerns, offering a natural and personalized approach to skincare. The aromas of the oils add to the sensory experience and the overall therapeutic effect, making topical application a holistic method for both physical and emotional wellness.

Essential Oils in Household Products

The integration of essential oils into household products is a growing trend, reflecting a shift towards more natural and eco-friendly cleaning solutions. Essential oils are valued for their pleasant, natural fragrances and their antibacterial and antiseptic properties, making them an ideal addition to homemade or commercial cleaning products. For instance, lemon and orange oils are popular for their fresh, invigorating scents and grease-cutting capabilities, ideal for kitchen cleaners. Tea tree and eucalyptus oils are known for their potent antimicrobial properties, making them suitable for disinfecting surfaces. Lavender, with its calming scent, is excellent for laundry detergents or fabric refreshers.

Adding these oils to cleaning agents not only enhances the cleaning power but also infuses the home with natural aromas, creating a pleasant and toxin-free environment. Furthermore, their use in household products aligns with a growing preference for products that are safe for both the environment and the family, steering away from harsh chemicals and synthetic fragrances.

Natural Remedies

The use of essential oils as natural remedies is an age-old practice, with various oils being celebrated for their specific health benefits. Peppermint oil, for instance, is widely recognized for aiding digestion and relieving symptoms of irritable bowel syndrome, thanks to its soothing properties on the gastrointestinal tract. It is also a popular choice for alleviating headaches and boosting energy levels. Lavender oil, known for its calming and sedative properties, is frequently used to promote relaxation, reduce anxiety, and improve sleep quality. Eucalyptus oil is often used for its respiratory benefits, helping to clear nasal congestion and relieve symptoms of colds and coughs.

These essential oils are used in various forms, such as inhaled through diffusers, applied topically when diluted with a carrier oil, or added to baths. It is important to note that while essential oils can offer significant health benefits, they are complementary treatments and should be used in conjunction with, rather than as a replacement for, traditional medical care. Moreover, individual responses to essential oils can vary, so it is advisable to start with small doses and observe how one's body reacts.

The multifaceted use of essential oils underscores their versatility and the growing interest in natural, plant-based solutions for health and lifestyle needs.

4

Safety First

Skin Sensitivity

The use of essential oils requires careful consideration due to the potential for skin sensitivity, which can lead to allergic reactions or irritation in some individuals. The highly concentrated nature of these oils means that they can be quite potent, and when applied directly to the skin, they may cause adverse reactions such as redness, itching, or rash. This sensitivity varies from person to person and can depend on the specific oil being used. Some oils are known to be more irritative than others, especially for those with sensitive skin or existing skin conditions.

To mitigate these risks, it is recommended to always perform a patch test before using a new essential oil and to dilute the oil with a carrier oil, such as almond or olive oil (and many more), to lessen its intensity. This practice helps in safely reaping the benefits of essential oils while minimizing the likelihood of skin-related issues.

It is also important for individuals to familiarize themselves with the properties of different oils and to seek advice from a healthcare professional, especially if they have a history of skin sensitivity or allergies.

Quality and Purity

In the realm of essential oils, the quality and purity of the product are paramount, especially for therapeutic use. The market for essential oils is diverse, with a significant variation in quality among different brands and products. High-quality, pure, unadulterated oils are the gold standard, as they ensure the most effective and safe experience.

Pure oils contain no synthetic additives or diluents and maintain the integrity of the plant's original chemical composition. The presence of impurities or additives can diminish the therapeutic properties of the oils and potentially lead to adverse effects. Therefore, it is crucial for users to diligently research and select reputable brands that provide transparent information about their sourcing, extraction methods, and testing protocols. This careful selection ensures that the oils are as close to their natural state as possible, offering the full spectrum of their benefits.

For individuals seeking to integrate essential oils into their wellness routine, investing in high-quality, pure oils is a critical step towards ensuring both efficacy and safety.

Ingestion

When it comes to the ingestion of essential oils, exercising caution is crucial. Generally, it is not recommended to consume these oils without the guidance of a qualified professional, such as an aromatherapist or healthcare provider. Essential oils are highly concentrated substances, and their ingestion can lead to toxicity or adverse reactions, particularly if used improperly or in excessive amounts.

The internal use of essential oils can affect organs and systems within the body, and risks may include gastrointestinal upset, liver damage, and harmful interactions with medications. The safety of ingesting essential oils varies depending on the specific oil, the individual's health, and the dosage. Therefore, any consideration of oral use should be based on a thorough understanding of the oil's properties and potential effects, alongside professional advice. This cautious approach is key to ensuring the safe and effective use of essential oils, particularly in a therapeutic context.

When to Consult a Healthcare Professional

When integrating essential oils into a health and wellness routine, consulting healthcare providers is a critical step, particularly for individuals who are pregnant, nursing, or have existing health conditions. Essential oils, with their potent and bioactive compounds, can have significant physiological effects. For pregnant women, certain oils can pose risks to the developing fetus or affect the pregnancy itself. Similarly, nursing mothers need to be cautious as some components of essential oils can be transferred to the baby through breast milk.

Individuals with pre-existing health conditions, such as epilepsy, high blood pressure, or asthma, may find that some oils exacerbate their symptoms or interact with their medications. A healthcare provider, knowledgeable about the individual's medical history and current health status, can offer personalized advice on how to incorporate essential oils into their wellness routine. Overall, by adhering to these safety guidelines, individuals can enjoy the benefits of essential oils while minimizing potential risks.

5

Storing Essential Oils

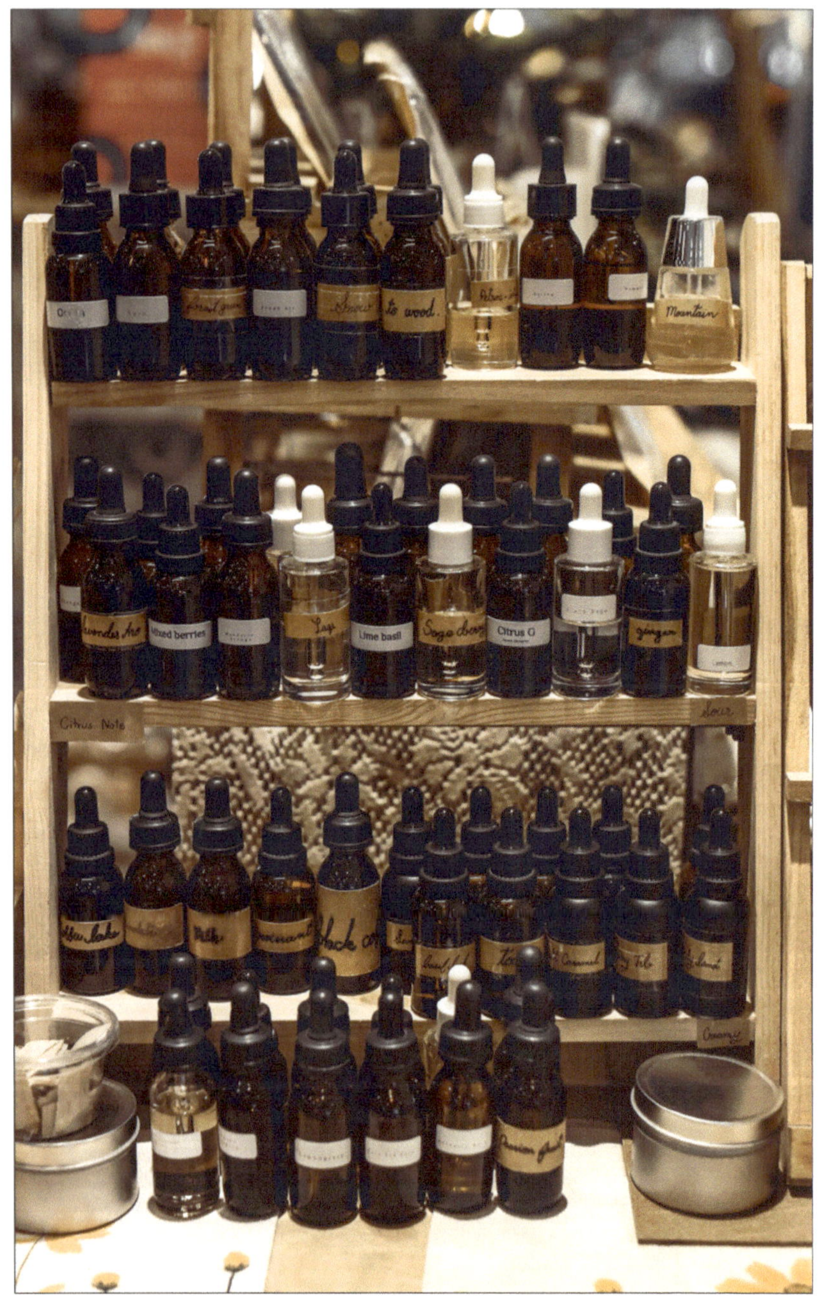

Proper storage of essential oils is crucial to maintaining their efficacy and longevity. They should ideally be kept in a cool, dark place, away from direct sunlight and fluctuating temperatures. Exposure to heat and light can lead to the degradation of the oils, altering their chemical composition and diminishing their therapeutic qualities.

Dark-colored glass bottles, such as amber or cobalt blue, are preferred for storage as they help block out damaging light. Additionally, most essential oils have a shelf life of approximately 1-3 years. However, this varies depending on the type of oil. For instance, citrus oils typically have a shorter shelf life due to their more volatile nature, often around 1-2 years, whereas heavier, more stable oils like sandalwood or patchouli can last longer, sometimes up to 4-6 years.

It is important to note that exposure to air, light, and heat can accelerate the deterioration process, so keeping the lids tightly closed and avoiding unnecessary exposure to air is also crucial. To extend their shelf life, some people store their oils in the refrigerator, although this is not necessary for all types. Properly storing essential oils ensures that their aromatic and therapeutic properties are preserved, allowing for effective use throughout their lifespan.

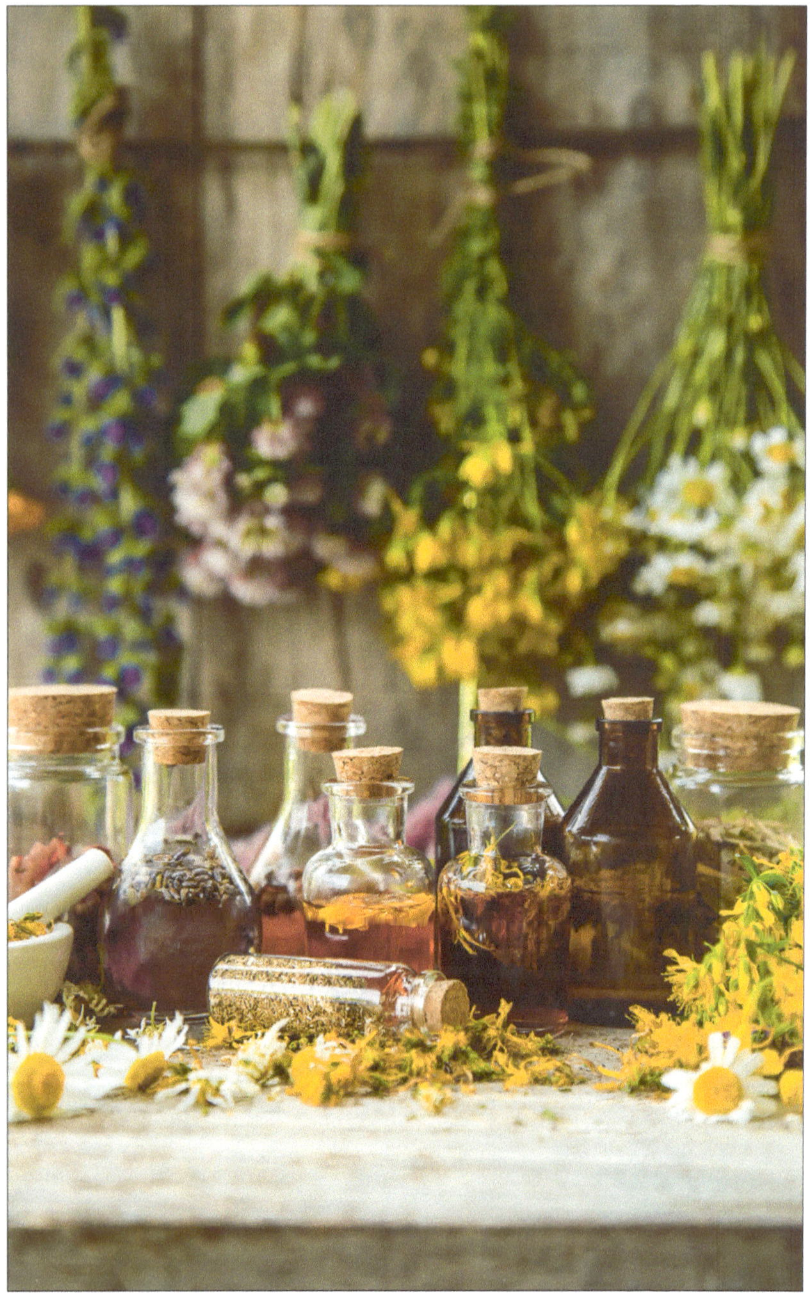

6

My Top 10 Essential Oils

The popularity of essential oils often depends on their versatility, therapeutic properties, and pleasant aromas. In this guide, we will cover my top ten essential oils, which are listed below.

1. Lavender
2. Peppermint
3. Tea Tree
4. Eucalyptus
5. Lemon
6. Frankincense
7. Chamomile
8. Rosemary
9. Ylang Ylang
10. Sandalwood

Each of these oils have different properties and compositions that offer unique benefits, contributing to their popularity in various applications, from aromatherapy and natural remedies to skincare and household cleaning products. Their widespread use is a testament to the growing interest in natural, plant-based solutions for health and wellness.

While essential oils offer various health benefits, they are not substitutes for professional medical advice or treatment. If you're considering using them for therapeutic purposes, especially if you have pre-existing health conditions or are on medication, consulting with a healthcare provider is highly advisable.

7

₂₃

Lavender

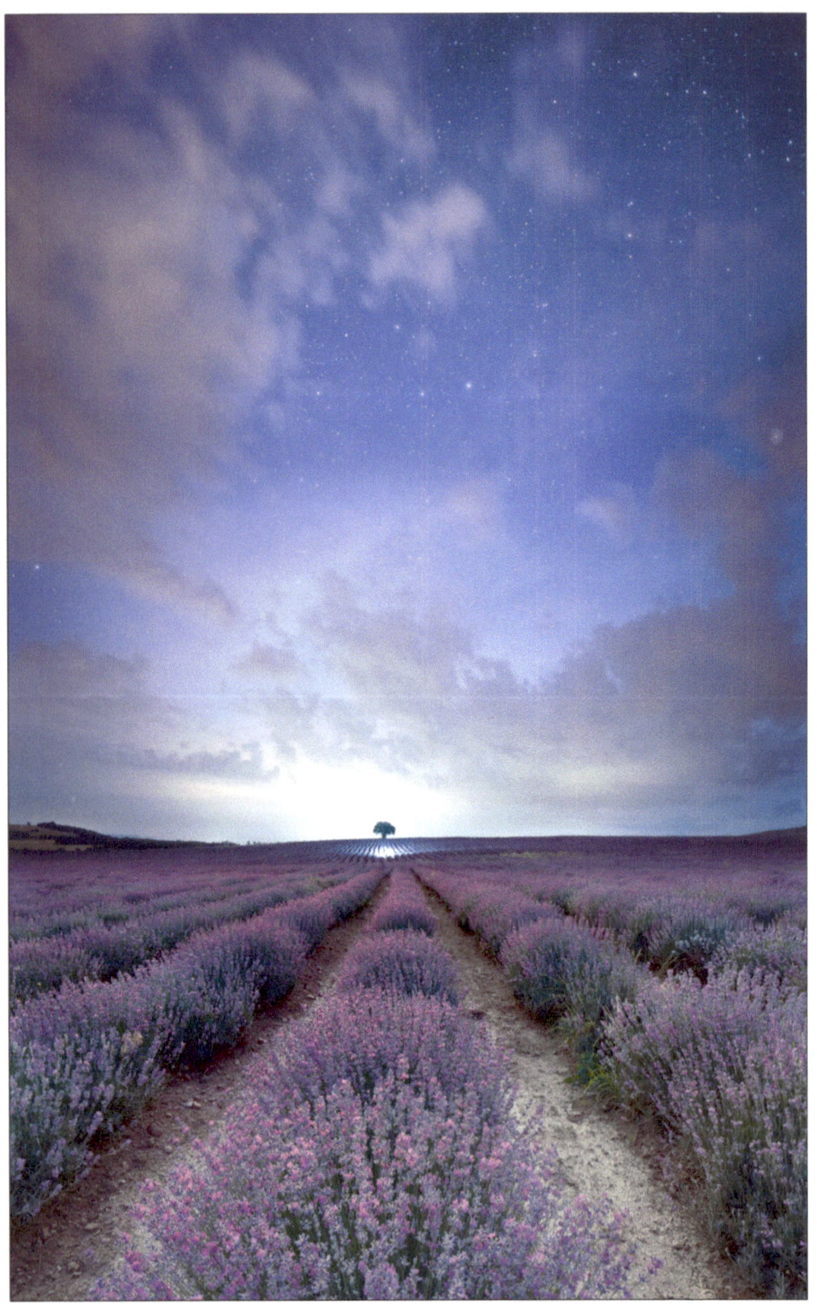

Lavender, known botanically as Lavandula, is a popular plant known for its aromatic flowers and numerous beneficial properties.

Properties of Lavender

Aromatic Scent: Lavender is most famous for its calming and soothing fragrance, which is widely used in aromatherapy.

Color: Lavender flowers are typically a shade of purple, but they can also range from blue to violet.

Herbal Uses: It is commonly used in herbal medicine, either in dried form or as an essential oil.

Culinary Applications: The flowers and leaves can be used in culinary preparations, adding a floral, slightly sweet flavor to dishes.

Health Benefits of Lavender

Stress and Anxiety Relief: One of the most well-known benefits of lavender is its ability to reduce stress and anxiety. Inhalation of lavender essential oil is often used in aromatherapy to induce relaxation and alleviate anxiety symptoms.

Sleep Aid: Lavender is commonly used to improve sleep quality. Its soothing scent is believed to help with insomnia and other sleep disorders.

Anti-Inflammatory and Antiseptic Properties: Lavender oil has anti-inflammatory and antiseptic properties, which can be beneficial in healing minor burns, insect bites, and acne.

Pain Relief: It can provide relief from pain, especially headaches, migraines, or muscle aches and tensions when used in massages or aromatherapy.

Digestive Health: Lavender may help in treating various digestive issues such as bloating, nausea, and upset stomach.

Skin Care: Due to its antiseptic and anti-inflammatory properties, lavender is often included in skin care products. It can help in treating and soothing various skin conditions like eczema, psoriasis, and acne.

Respiratory Health: Inhaling lavender steam or using lavender essential oil in a diffuser can help clear the nasal passage and relieve symptoms of colds, flu, asthma, and allergies.

Precautions

While lavender is generally safe for most people, it is important to use it correctly, especially when dealing with essential oils. Some individuals may experience allergic reactions, and it is advised to do a patch test before using it extensively on the skin. Also, pregnant or breastfeeding women should consult a healthcare professional before using lavender as a treatment.

8

Peppermint

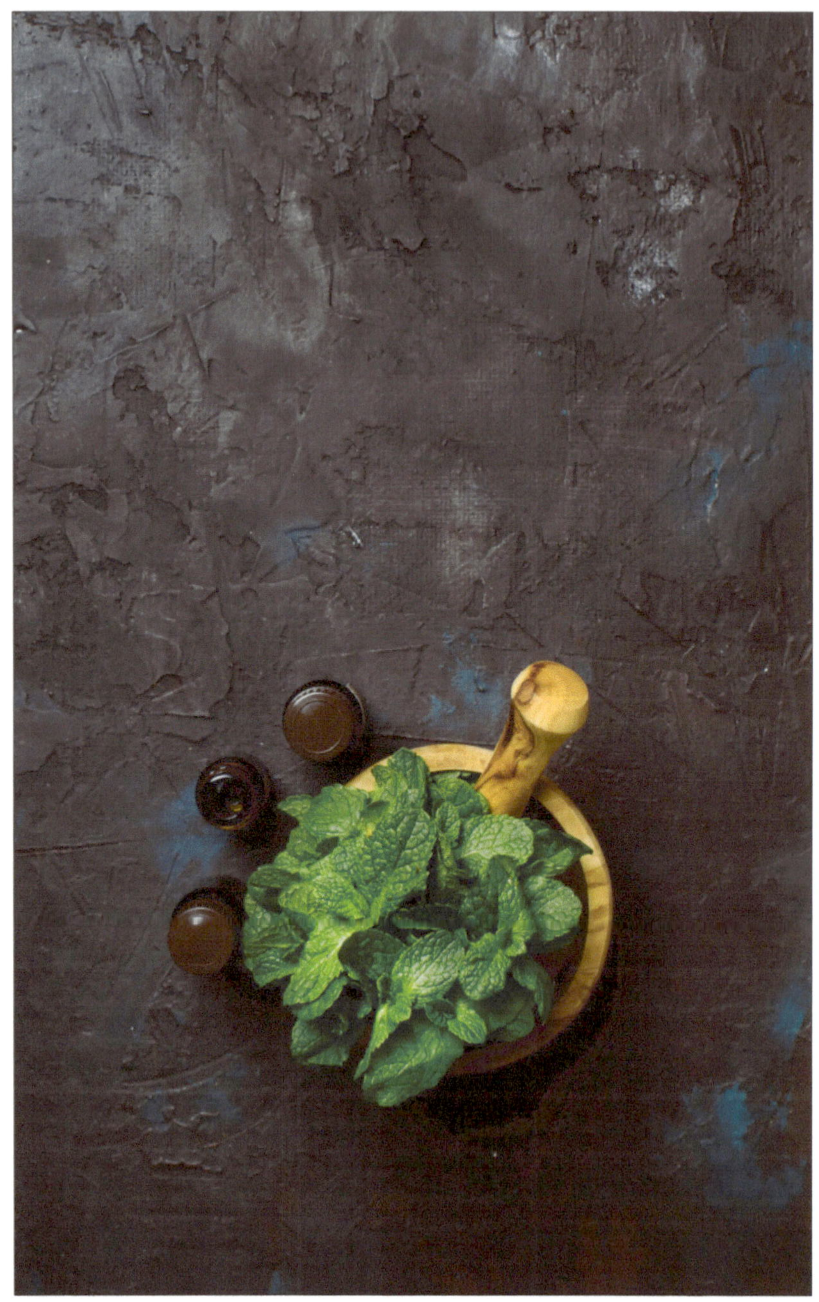

Peppermint, known scientifically as Mentha piperita, is a popular herb renowned for its distinctive aroma and numerous health benefits.

Properties of Peppermint

Aroma: Peppermint is known for its strong, refreshing, and cool aroma, which comes from its high menthol content.

Appearance: It typically has dark green leaves and sometimes features small, purple flowers.

Taste: The flavor is intensely minty, often described as a blend of sweetness and sharp, cooling sensation.

Cultivation: It is a hybrid mint, a cross between watermint and spearmint, widely cultivated in Europe and North America.

Uses: Peppermint is used in various forms—leaves (fresh or dried), essential oil, extracts, and teas. It is common in culinary, medicinal, and cosmetic applications.

Health Benefits of Peppermint

Digestive Health: Peppermint is well-known for its ability to soothe digestive issues. It can help relieve symptoms of irritable bowel syndrome (IBS), including bloating, gas, and intestinal spasms.

Pain Relief: Applied topically, peppermint oil can help relieve pain. It is often used in balms and ointments to soothe muscle aches, headaches, and even nerve pain.

<u>Nasal and Respiratory Benefits</u>: The menthol in peppermint acts as a decongestant, helping to clear the respiratory tract. It is beneficial in relieving coughs, colds, sinusitis, asthma, and bronchitis.

<u>Oral Health</u>: Peppermint is antibacterial and antifungal, making it effective in improving oral health. It is commonly found in toothpaste and mouthwashes to freshen breath and reduce dental plaque.

<u>Nausea Relief</u>: The aroma of peppermint oil can help reduce nausea, making it a helpful natural remedy for morning sickness or motion sickness.

<u>Mental Performance and Alertness</u>: Inhaling peppermint aroma can improve mental alertness and cognitive function, making it a popular choice for diffusing in study or work environments.

<u>Skin Health</u>: Peppermint oil has cooling and soothing properties for the skin. It is used to relieve itching, inflammation, and sunburn.

Precautions

While peppermint is generally safe for most people, it is important to use it correctly. Peppermint oil should be diluted before topical application, and some people might experience allergic reactions. Ingesting high concentrations of peppermint oil can be toxic, so it should be used with caution. People with gastroesophageal reflux disease (GERD) or hiatal hernia should avoid peppermint, as it can exacerbate these conditions. Pregnant or breastfeeding women should consult a healthcare provider before using peppermint in medicinal forms.

9

Tea Tree

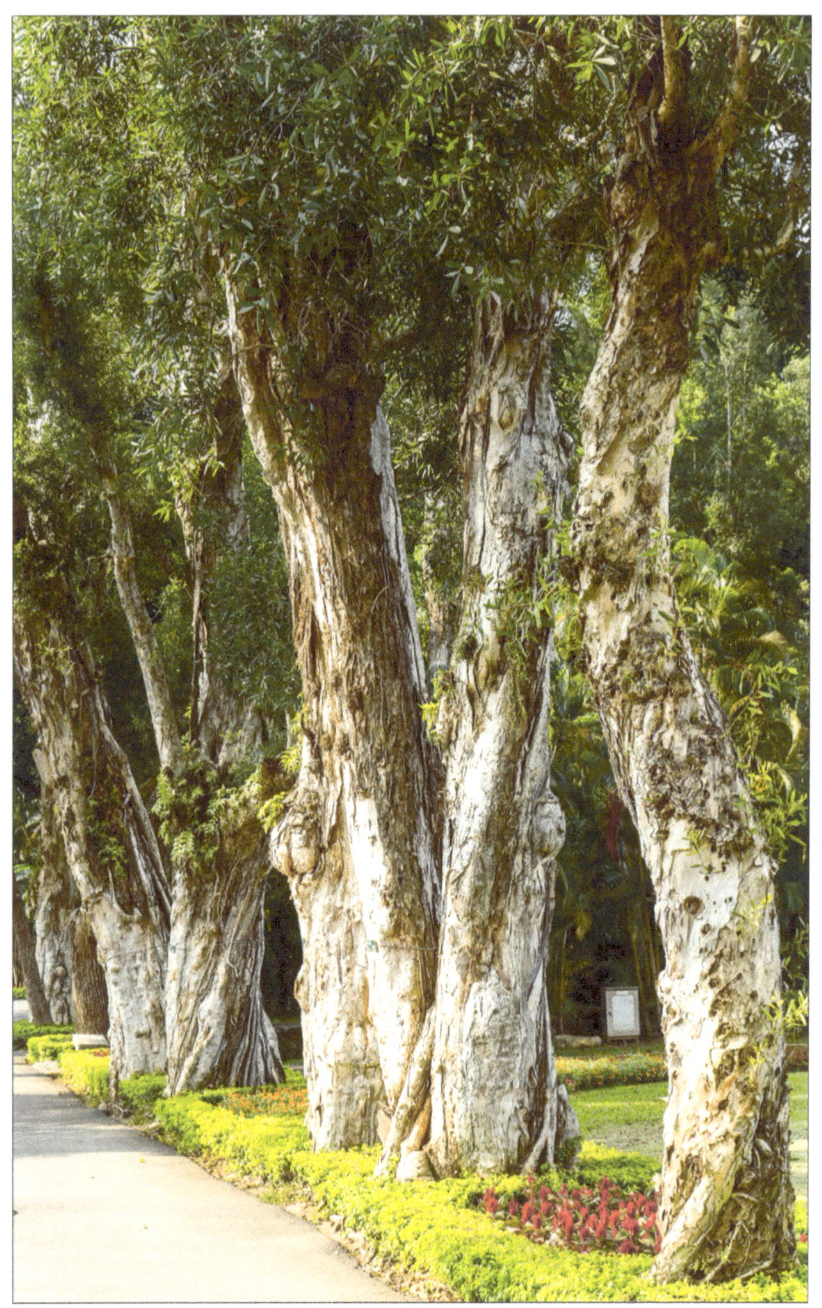

Tea tree oil, derived from the leaves of the Melaleuca alternifolia tree native to Australia, is known for its distinctive properties and a wide range of health benefits. It is important to note that tea tree oil is typically used topically (applied to the skin) and should not be ingested.

Properties of Tea Tree Oil

Antimicrobial: It possesses strong antibacterial, antiviral, and antifungal properties, making it effective against various pathogens.

Aroma: Tea tree oil has a fresh, camphoraceous smell, which is sharp and slightly medicinal.

Appearance: The oil is clear to pale yellow in color.

Solubility: It is not soluble in water but can be diluted in carrier oils, creams, or lotions.

Health Benefits of Tea Tree Oil

Skin Health: Tea tree oil is renowned for its ability to treat various skin conditions. It is effective in managing acne, reducing inflammation, and aiding in wound healing.

Antifungal Properties: Due to its antifungal properties, it is often used to treat fungal infections like athlete's foot, nail fungus, and ringworm.

Hair and Scalp Treatment: It can help in treating dandruff, lice, and other scalp conditions, owing to its antimicrobial properties and ability to soothe the scalp.

Oral Health: When used in mouthwash (but not swallowed), it can help combat bad breath and dental plaque, thanks to its antibacterial properties.

Anti-Inflammatory: Tea tree oil's anti-inflammatory effects can provide relief from skin irritations and insect bites.

Immune System Support: Its antimicrobial properties may help in strengthening the body's defense against various pathogens.

Aromatherapy: In aromatherapy, tea tree oil is used for its potential to cleanse, purify, and rejuvenate the mind and body.

Precautions and Usage Tips

Topical Use Only: Tea tree oil is toxic if swallowed.

Dilution: It should be diluted with a carrier oil (like coconut or almond oil) before applying to the skin, especially for those with sensitive skin.

Patch Test: Conduct a patch test to check for an allergic reaction.

Avoid Contact with Eyes and Mucous Membranes: It can be irritating if it gets into the eyes or is applied to mucous membranes.

Pregnancy and Breastfeeding: Caution is advised for pregnant or breastfeeding women. Consult a physician.

Children and Pets: Be cautious when using around children and pets, as they can be more sensitive to the effects of essential oils.

10

Eucalyptus

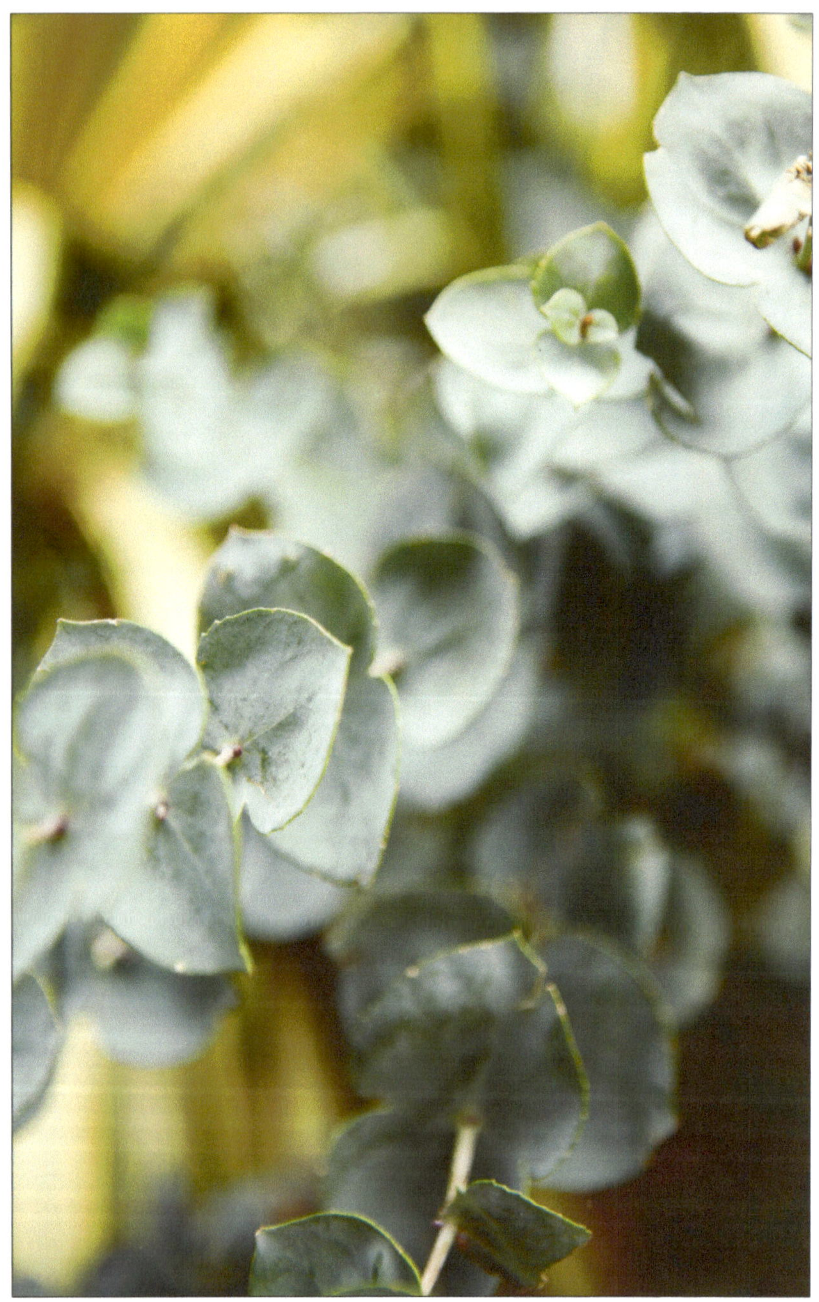

Eucalyptus, derived from the leaves of the eucalyptus tree, is known for its potent properties and a range of health benefits. Eucalyptus oil, in particular, is widely used for its therapeutic qualities.

Properties of Eucalyptus

Aroma: Eucalyptus oil has a distinctively fresh, sharp, and clean scent, often described as camphoraceous with a hint of sweetness.

Chemical Composition: The primary component is 1,8-cineole, also known as eucalyptol, which contributes to its medicinal properties.

Appearance: Eucalyptus oil is typically clear in color.

Texture: It is relatively thin in consistency.

Health Benefits of Eucalyptus

Respiratory Health: One of the most recognized benefits of eucalyptus is its ability to aid respiratory health. It can help relieve symptoms of coughs, colds, sinusitis, asthma, and bronchitis. The eucalyptol in eucalyptus oil helps to break up mucus and has decongestant properties.

Pain Relief: Eucalyptus oil is often used in ointments and creams to relieve muscle and joint pain. Its anti-inflammatory properties can help reduce pain and inflammation.

Antimicrobial Properties: Eucalyptus oil has antibacterial, antifungal, and antiviral properties, making it useful in treating infections and as a natural disinfectant.

Mental Clarity: The refreshing aroma of eucalyptus oil can promote mental clarity and reduce stress. It is often used in aromatherapy for stimulating mental activity and increasing blood flow to the brain.

Skin Care: Due to its antimicrobial and anti-inflammatory properties, eucalyptus oil can be beneficial for skin care, especially in treating acne, wounds, and minor burns.

Dental Health: Eucalyptus oil is also known for its ability to fight bacteria that cause tooth decay and periodontitis, making it a component in some mouthwashes and dental preparations.

Insect Repellent: Its strong scent is effective in repelling mosquitoes and other insects. It is often used in natural insect repellent products.

Precautions and Usage Tips

Dilution for Topical Use: Eucalyptus oil should be diluted with a carrier oil before applying to the skin.

Inhalation: It can be inhaled directly or used in a diffuser for respiratory benefits or aromatherapy.

Avoid Ingestion: Eucalyptus oil should not be ingested as it can be toxic.

Patch Test: Do a patch test to check for allergic reactions.

Pregnancy and Breastfeeding: Consult a healthcare provider before use during pregnancy and breastfeeding.

Children and Pets: Use with caution around children and pets.

11

Lemon

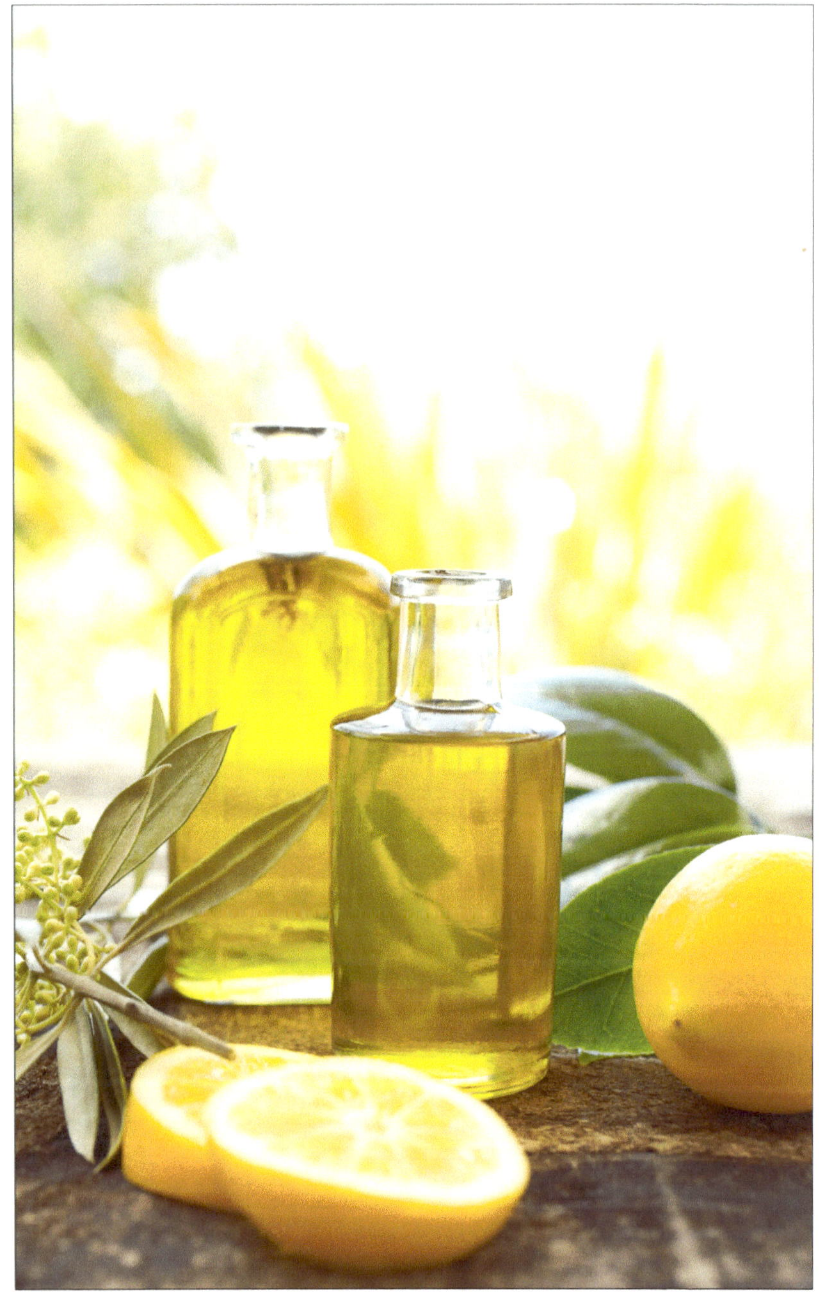

Lemon essential oil, extracted from the peel of the lemon fruit (Citrus limon), is celebrated for its refreshing scent and a multitude of health benefits.

Properties of Lemon Essential Oil

Aroma: Lemon essential oil is known for its clean, sharp, and refreshing citrus scent. It is often used to invigorate and uplift the mood.

Appearance: The oil is usually a pale-yellow color.

Chemical Composition: It is rich in limonene, which contributes to its aromatic and therapeutic properties.

Solubility: Like most essential oils, it is not water-soluble but can be diluted in carrier oils or alcohol.

Health Benefits of Lemon Essential Oil

Mood Enhancement: The uplifting aroma of lemon essential oil can help improve mood and reduce symptoms of anxiety and depression.

Antimicrobial Properties: It has strong antibacterial and antiviral properties, making it effective in disinfecting and cleaning. It is often used in homemade cleaning products for this reason.

Digestive Health: Lemon oil can help alleviate digestive problems when used in aromatherapy. It is known to relieve nausea, especially related to pregnancy or motion sickness.

Skin Care: When diluted and applied topically, lemon essential oil can improve skin health. It is known for its astringent properties and ability to cleanse skin, reduce acne, and even brighten the complexion.

Respiratory Health: Inhaling lemon oil can help clear nasal passages and relieve symptoms of coughs and colds.

Boosting Immune System: Lemon essential oil is rich in vitamins and antioxidants, which can help boost the immune system.

Relief from Stress and Anxiety: Its refreshing scent is known to reduce stress and anxiety when used in aromatherapy.

Precautions and Usage Tips

Skin Sensitivity and Photosensitivity: Lemon oil can make the skin more sensitive to sunlight, leading to increased risk of sunburn. It is advised to avoid sun exposure for several hours after applying it to the skin.

Dilution for Topical Use: Always dilute lemon essential oil with a carrier oil before applying it to the skin to avoid irritation.

Internal Use Caution: Ingesting lemon essential oil is generally not recommended without the guidance of a healthcare professional.

Allergy Test: Conduct a patch test before widespread use to ensure you do not have an allergic reaction.

Storage: Store it in a dark, cool place to maintain its potency.

12

Frankincense

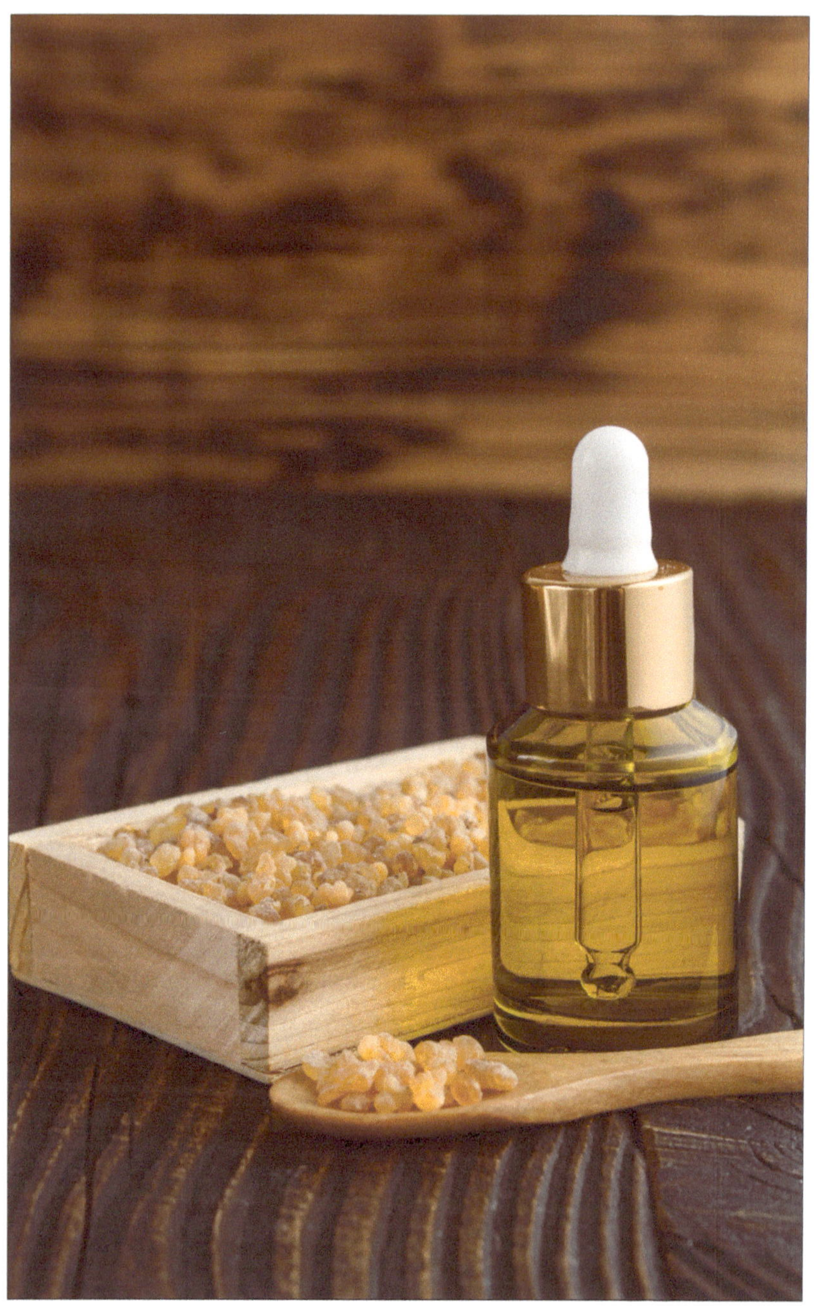

Frankincense oil, derived from the resin of the Boswellia tree species, has been valued for centuries for its aromatic and therapeutic properties.

Properties of Frankincense Oil

Aroma: Frankincense oil has a distinctive woody, spicy, and slightly fruity aroma with a calming and grounding effect.

Chemical Composition: It contains compounds like alpha-pinene, limonene, and incensole, which contribute to its therapeutic effects.

Appearance: The oil is generally a pale yellow or greenish color.

Texture: It has a relatively thin consistency.

Health Benefits of Frankincense Oil

Stress and Anxiety Reduction: Frankincense oil is known for its ability to promote relaxation and tranquility. It is often used in aromatherapy to reduce feelings of stress and anxiety.

Anti-Inflammatory Properties: The oil has anti-inflammatory effects, which can help reduce joint inflammation and assist in conditions like arthritis.

Immune System Support: Frankincense is believed to boost the immune system. Its antiseptic properties can help prevent the development and spread of harmful microorganisms.

Skin Health: Frankincense oil is beneficial for skin health, known to promote the healing of scars, wounds, and stretch marks, as well as to reduce the appearance of wrinkles and age spots.

Respiratory Benefits: It can help relieve congestion and promote easier breathing, making it a useful remedy for respiratory conditions like asthma or bronchitis.

Digestive Health: In traditional medicine, frankincense has been used to improve digestion and to relieve symptoms of gastrointestinal discomfort.

Mental Focus and Cognitive Function: The oil is often used in aromatherapy to enhance focus, concentration, and mental clarity.

Precautions and Usage Tips

Dilution for Topical Use: Frankincense oil should be diluted with a carrier oil before applying to the skin.

Allergy Test: Conduct a patch test before using it extensively, to ensure there is no allergic reaction.

Pregnancy and Breastfeeding: Caution is advised for pregnant or breastfeeding women. Consult a healthcare provider before use.

Internal Use: Generally, it is not recommended to ingest Frankincense oil.

Interactions with Medications: If you are on medication, especially those related to blood-thinning or for managing blood pressure, consult a healthcare provider before using frankincense oil.

13

Chamomile

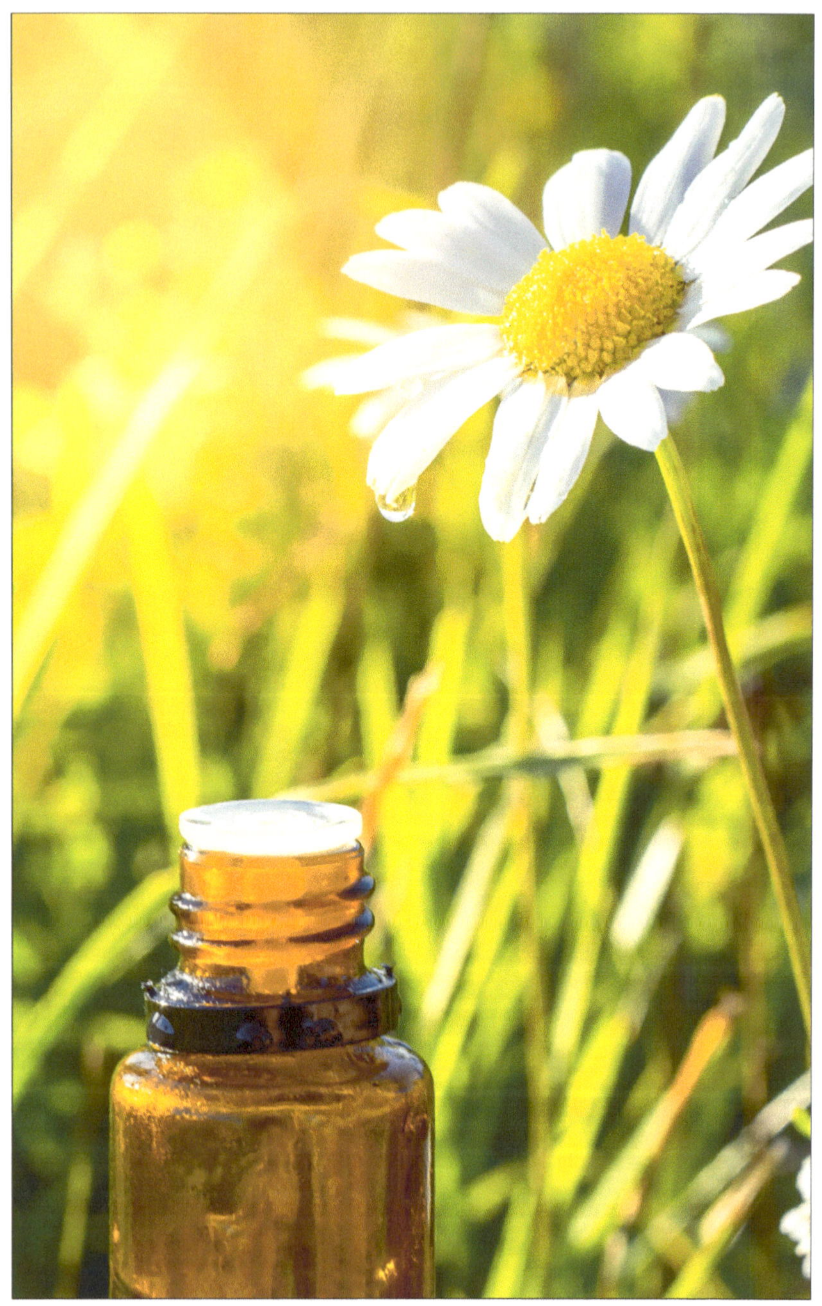

Chamomile oil, derived from the flowers of the chamomile plant (commonly either Roman Chamomile or German Chamomile), is renowned for its therapeutic properties and a multitude of health benefits.

Properties of Chamomile Oil

Aroma: Chamomile oil typically has a sweet, floral, and herbaceous aroma. It is known for its calming and soothing scent.

Chemical Composition: It contains compounds like bisabolol, chamazulene, and flavonoids, which contribute to its therapeutic properties.

Appearance: The color can range from clear to a deep blue, depending on the type of chamomile and the extraction process.

Texture: It has a medium to viscous consistency.

Health Benefits of Chamomile Oil

Stress and Anxiety Relief: Chamomile oil is widely used in aromatherapy for its ability to calm the mind and reduce anxiety. It is often used to promote relaxation and improve sleep quality.

Anti-Inflammatory and Pain Relief: Its notable anti-inflammatory properties make it beneficial in reducing pain and inflammation, especially in conditions like arthritis, back pain, and neuralgia.

Skin Health: Chamomile oil is gentle on the skin and is known for its ability to soothe irritated skin, reduce redness, and support the healing of conditions like eczema, acne, and sunburn.

Digestive Health: It can soothe the digestive system and is often used to relieve gastrointestinal issues like gas, indigestion, and nausea.

Wound Healing: Due to its antiseptic and anti-inflammatory properties, chamomile oil can promote faster healing of minor wounds, cuts, and bruises.

Sedative Properties: Its mild sedative effects make it a useful aid for those suffering from insomnia or having trouble sleeping.

Respiratory Health: When inhaled, chamomile oil can help in relieving symptoms of colds, allergies, and sinus issues.

Precautions and Usage Tips

Dilution: Chamomile oil should be diluted with a carrier oil before applying to the skin.

Allergy Test: Conduct a patch test before using extensively, especially if you have allergies to plants in the Asteraceae family.

Pregnancy and Breastfeeding: Caution is advised during pregnancy and breastfeeding. Consult a healthcare provider before use.

Internal Use: It is generally not recommended to ingest Chamomile essential oil.

Interactions with Medications: Chamomile oil can interact with certain medications (i.e., blood thinners). Consult a healthcare provider.

14

Rosemary

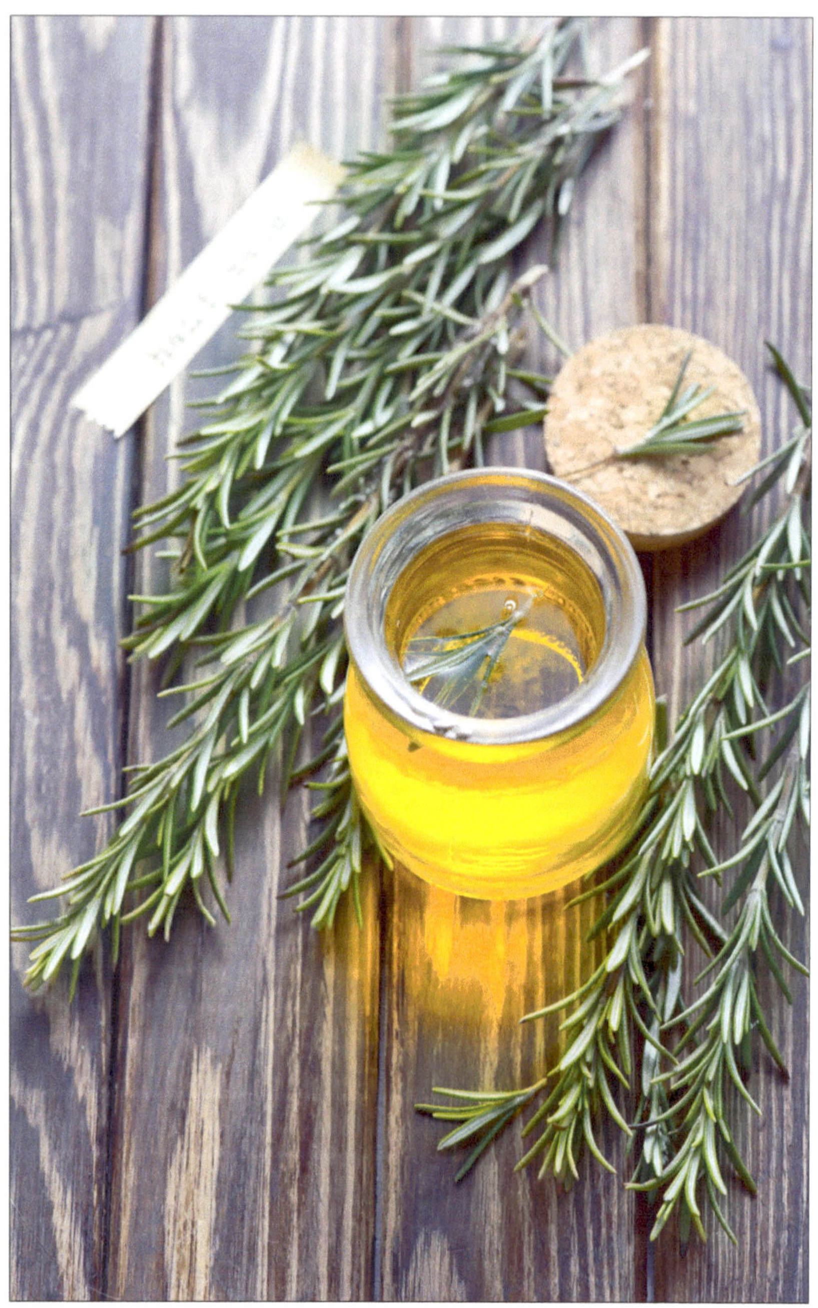

Rosemary oil, extracted from the leaves of the Rosmarinus officinalis plant, is known for its distinctive aroma and a wide range of health benefits. It is a versatile oil used in various applications, from culinary to cosmetic and medicinal.

Properties of Rosemary Oil

Aroma: Rosemary oil has a strong, fresh, woody, and herbal scent. It is known for its invigorating and stimulating aroma.

Chemical Composition: Key components include cineole, camphor, and alpha-pinene, which contribute to its therapeutic properties.

Appearance: The oil is generally clear to pale yellow in color.

Texture: It has a watery viscosity.

Health Benefits of Rosemary Oil

Cognitive Function: Rosemary oil is reputed to enhance cognitive function, improving concentration, focus, and memory. It is often used in aromatherapy for mental clarity.

Hair Health: It is popular in hair care for promoting hair growth, reducing dandruff, and strengthening the hair.

Pain Relief: The oil has analgesic properties, making it effective in relieving muscle aches, joint pain, and headaches.

Stress Relief: The refreshing aroma of rosemary oil can help alleviate stress and anxiety, promoting a sense of well-being.

Antimicrobial Properties: Rosemary oil has antimicrobial and antiseptic qualities, making it useful in treating various skin conditions and in natural cleaning solutions.

Respiratory Health: Its anti-inflammatory and antispasmodic properties can help relieve asthma, bronchitis, and sinusitis.

Digestive Health: Rosemary oil can aid in digestion and help relieve digestive problems like indigestion, gas, and bloating.

Immune System Support: The oil is known for its ability to boost the immune system, potentially helping to fend off infections.

Precautions and Usage Tips

Dilution for Topical Use: Always dilute rosemary oil with a carrier oil before applying it to the skin to prevent irritation.

Avoid During Pregnancy: Rosemary oil is not recommended for use during pregnancy.

Epilepsy and High Blood Pressure: Individuals with epilepsy or high blood pressure should use caution, as the oil can be stimulating.

Allergy Test: Conduct a patch test to check for allergic reactions.

Internal Use Caution: Rosemary essential oil should not be ingested.

Children and Pets: Use with caution around children and pets.

15

Ylang Ylang

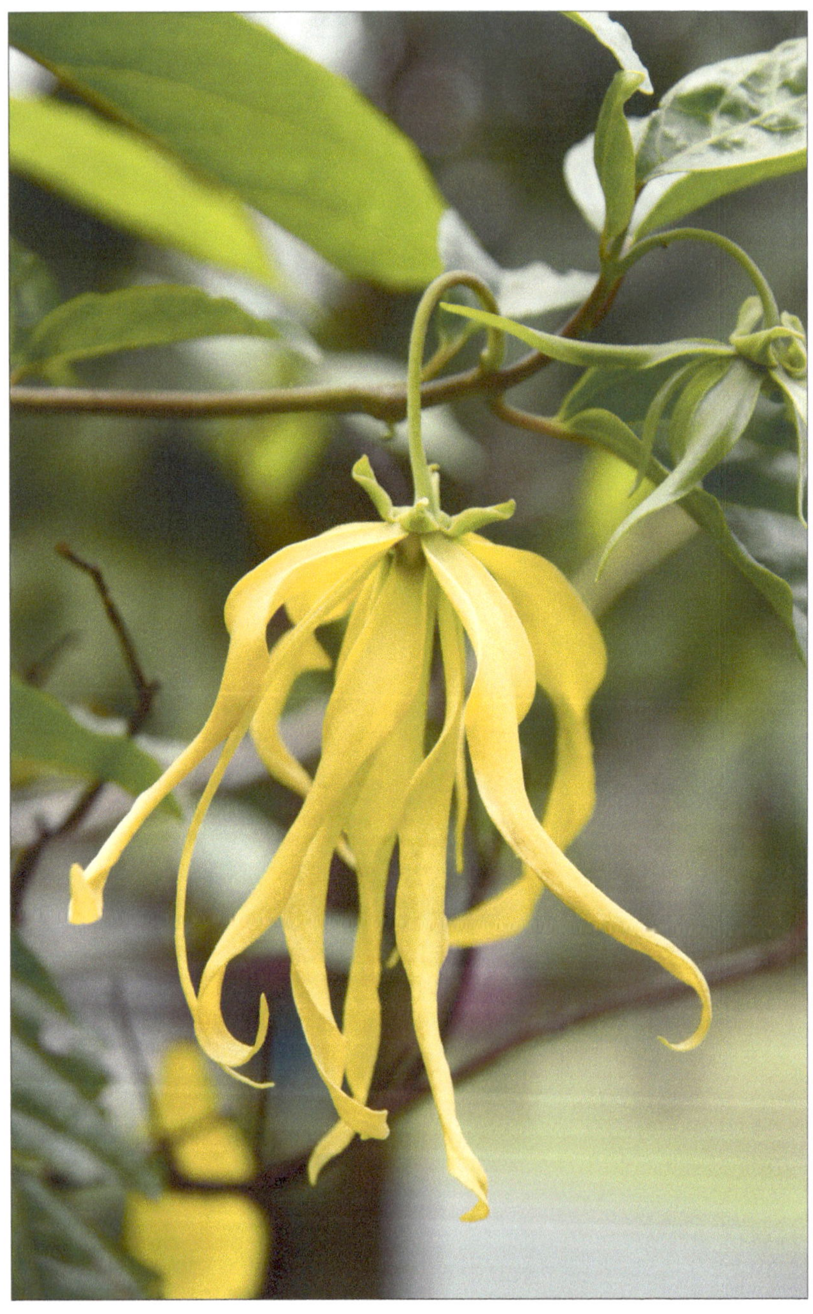

Ylang Ylang oil, extracted from the flowers of the Cananga odorata tree, is celebrated for its unique fragrance and various health benefits. Known for its use in perfumery and aromatherapy, this essential oil offers several therapeutic properties.

Properties of Ylang Ylang Oil

Aroma: Ylang Ylang oil has a rich, floral, and slightly fruity scent. It is sweet and exotic, creating a feeling of relaxation and euphoria.

Chemical Composition: Compounds like linalool, caryophyllene, and geranyl acetate, which contribute to its aroma and therapeutic benefits.

Appearance: The oil typically ranges from a pale to rich yellow color.

Texture: It has a fairly light consistency, not being too viscous.

Health Benefits of Ylang Ylang Oil

Stress and Anxiety Relief: The oil is well-regarded for its ability to reduce stress and anxiety levels, promoting a sense of calmness and relaxation. It is frequently used in aromatherapy for this purpose.

Mood Enhancement: Ylang Ylang can have uplifting effects on mood, often used to alleviate depression and enhance the mood.

Skin Health: Due to its antiseptic and nourishing properties, Ylang Ylang oil is beneficial for skin care, particularly in balancing oil production and improving skin tone.

Hair Health: It is often added to hair care products to promote shiny, healthy-looking hair and potentially stimulate hair growth.

Libido Boosting: Ylang Ylang oil has been used as an aphrodisiac believed to enhance sexual desire and improve intimate relationships.

Hypotensive Properties: It may help lower high blood pressure when used in moderation and in a controlled environment like aromatherapy.

Sedative Effects: It can have a mild sedative effect, aiding in reducing insomnia and promoting restful sleep.

Precautions and Usage Tips

Dilution for Topical Use: Ylang Ylang oil should be diluted with a carrier oil before applying to the skin to minimize the risk of irritation.

Patch Test: Conduct a patch test before extensive use to check for allergic reactions, especially if you have sensitive skin.

Moderation in Use: Due to its potent scent and effects, it should be used in moderation. Excessive use may lead to headaches or nausea.

Pregnancy and Breastfeeding: Consult a healthcare provider before using Ylang Ylang oil during pregnancy or breastfeeding.

Internal Use Caution: Ylang Ylang oil should not be ingested.

Interactions with Medication: If you are on medication, especially for blood pressure or sedatives, consult a healthcare provider before using.

16

Sandalwood

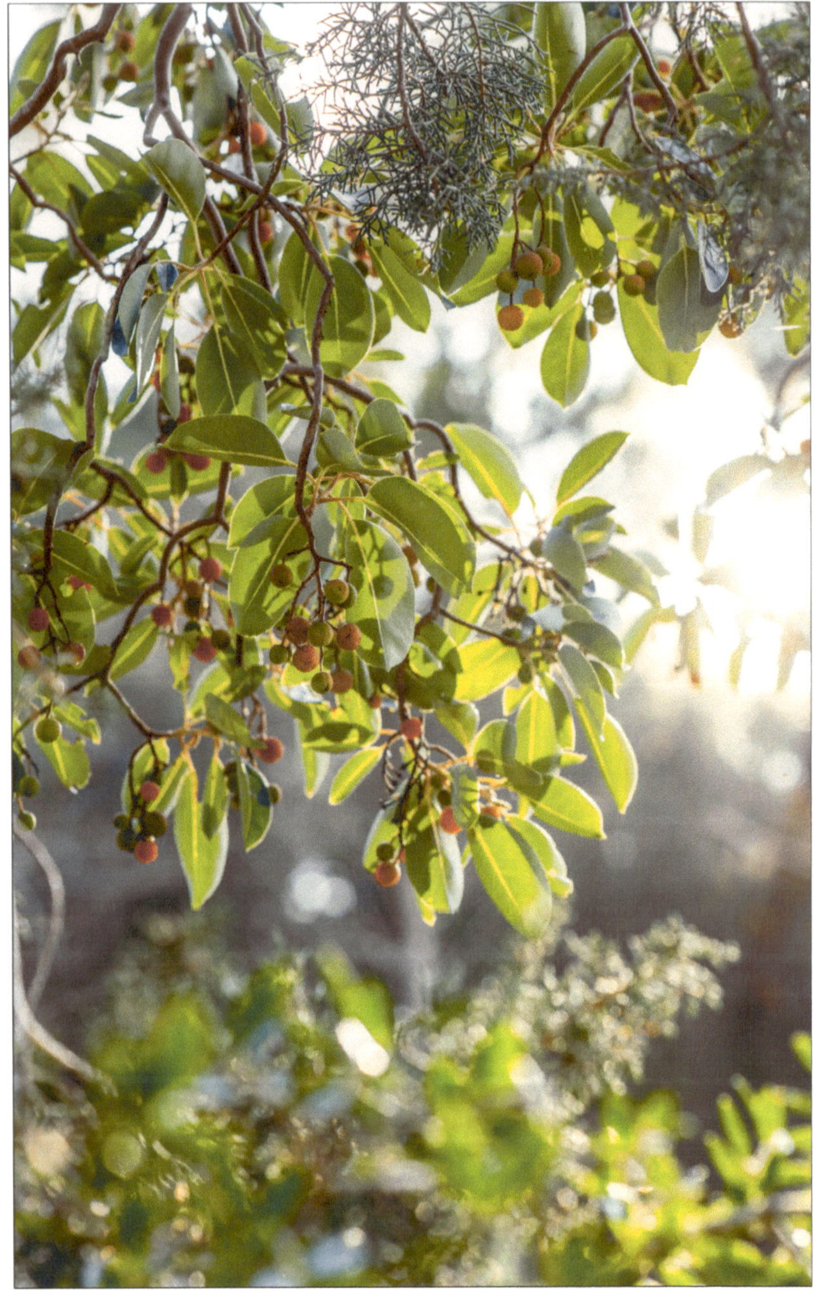

Sandalwood oil, derived from the wood and roots of the Santalum genus, is a highly valued essential oil known for its distinctive fragrance and therapeutic properties. It has been used traditionally in various cultural rituals and medicinal practices.

Properties of Sandalwood Oil

Aroma: Sandalwood oil has a rich, woody, earthy scent with subtle notes of sweetness. It is well-known for its calming and soothing aroma.

Chemical Composition: The primary component is santalol, which contributes to the oil's fragrance and therapeutic properties.

Appearance: The oil is typically a pale yellow to golden brown color.

Texture: It has a medium to viscous consistency.

Health Benefits of Sandalwood Oil

Mental Clarity and Relaxation: Sandalwood oil is often used in aromatherapy for its ability to promote mental clarity, calm the mind, and reduce stress and anxiety.

Skin Care: The oil is prized for its moisturizing and soothing properties. It is beneficial for treating dry skin, relieving itching, and reducing the appearance of scars and blemishes.

Anti-Inflammatory Properties: Sandalwood oil has anti-inflammatory effects, making it beneficial for soothing inflammation, such as in skin conditions or mild irritations.

Antiseptic and Antimicrobial: It has antiseptic properties, which can be helpful in preventing and treating infections when applied to the skin.

Sleep Aid: Its sedative properties can help improve sleep quality, making it a useful aid for those suffering from insomnia.

Respiratory Health: Inhaling sandalwood oil can have a soothing effect on the throat and may help in relieving coughs and sore throats.

Emotional Well-being: The oil is often used to promote emotional balance, reduce anxiety and stress, and enhance overall well-being.

Precautions and Usage Tips

Dilution: Sandalwood oil should be diluted with a carrier oil before topical application to prevent skin irritation.

Patch Test: Conduct a patch test before extensive use, especially for those with sensitive skin.

Pregnancy and Breastfeeding: Consult with a healthcare provider before using sandalwood oil during pregnancy or while breastfeeding.

Internal Use: Ingesting sandalwood oil is generally not recommended without professional guidance.

Cost and Sustainability: Pure sandalwood oil can be quite expensive. Also, due to overharvesting concerns, it is important to source the oil from sustainable and ethical producers.

17

Getting Started

Embarking on the journey of using essential oils can be both exciting and overwhelming due to the vast array of options and applications. To get started, it is advisable to begin small. Choose a few versatile oils, such as lavender, peppermint, and lemon, and familiarize yourself with their uses. This approach allows you to understand the basics without feeling overwhelmed.

Once comfortable, you can start experimenting with different combinations. Blending oils can not only create pleasant aromas but also enhance their therapeutic benefits. For instance, lavender and chamomile can be combined for relaxation, or peppermint and eucalyptus for a refreshing and clearing blend. However, it is important to remember that experimentation should be done mindfully, respecting safety guidelines, especially regarding skin application and diffusion.

Additionally, educating yourself is crucial in this journey. There are numerous resources available, including books, online articles, and workshops. These can provide valuable insights into the properties, uses, and safety considerations of various essential oils. Consulting with aromatherapy experts or healthcare professionals can also offer personalized guidance, especially when using essential oils for specific health concerns. This combination of starting small, experimenting, and seeking education forms a solid foundation for a safe and enjoyable experience with essential oils.

18

Finding Quality Oils

Finding quality essential oils is a critical step in ensuring you receive the full therapeutic benefits these oils can offer. It starts with identifying and choosing reputable brands, which can be achieved through thorough research and reading reviews from other users. Look for companies that are transparent about their sourcing, extraction methods, and quality testing procedures. These details are often indicators of the brand's commitment to providing pure and high-quality products.

Equally important is the need to avoid synthetic fragrances. Essential oils should be 100% pure, without any additives or synthetic substances. These pure oils offer the complete natural essence of the plant, including its therapeutic properties. Check labels carefully and beware of terms like "fragrance oil" or "perfume oil," as these are not true essential oils and often contain synthetic compounds. Labels that clearly state "100% essential oil" or provide GC/MS (Gas Chromatography/Mass Spectrometry) testing results are good indicators of quality. By prioritizing reputable brands and purity, you can ensure that the essential oils you select are not only effective, but also safe for use in aromatherapy, topical applications, and other uses.

19

10 Essential Oil Brands

Based on various sources, below is a list of some of the top essential oil brands listed in alphabetical order. There are many brands and the industry changes periodically, so it is important to do research to stay abreast of the latest developments. This is not intended to be an exhaustive list of the brands available on the market.

Aura Cacia: A company committed to high-quality, organic personal-care products, and known for its support of social and environmental responsibility.

doTERRA: Recognized for its pure essential oils sourced responsibly and its Certified Pure Tested Grade Protocols. They offer a vast range of essential oils, including rare types like rose oil.

Edens Garden: Offers a variety of high-quality, pure essential oils, and unique blends. They provide "Create Your Own Set" options and prioritize sustainable and ethical sourcing.

Jade Bloom Essential Oils: A brand known for its affordability and a wide range of products, including oils for sensitive skin, children, and the elderly.

Mountain Rose Herbs: Notable for supporting small-scale farmers and herbalists, emphasizing fair and sustainable sourcing practices, and offering a range of organic products.

Plant Therapy: Known for its third-party testing to ensure quality, offering a wide range of products including single oils, blends, roll-ons, and kid-safe options.

REVIVE Essential Oils: Appreciated for its quality, fair pricing, and fast shipping, they offer a variety of single oils, blends, and essential oil kits.

Rocky Mountain Oils: A brand with a focus on sourcing and quality assurance, known for its S.A.A.F.E Promise™ and offering a range of USDA Certified Organic oils.

Vitruvi: Offers all-natural essential oils with filler-free ingredient blends. They are also known for their popular diffusers and humidifiers.

Young Living: A well-established brand, recognized for its "Seed to Seal" process ensuring quality from planting to bottling, offering a range of products including single oils, blends, and diffusers.

These brands are recognized for their commitment to quality, purity, and sustainable practices. When choosing an essential oil brand, consider factors like third-party testing, sourcing, ethical practices, and customer reviews to ensure you are selecting a high-quality product.

20

Essential Oil Communities

Joining essential oil communities can be an enriching and educational part of your journey with essential oils. These communities, whether online forums, social media groups, or local clubs, offer a platform to connect with like-minded individuals who share an interest in aromatherapy and natural wellness. In these groups, members exchange tips, share experiences, and offer advice on using essential oils safely and effectively. It is a great way to stay updated on the latest trends, discover new uses for oils, and learn from the experiences of others.

For beginners, these communities can be particularly valuable, providing a supportive environment to ask questions and gain insights. More experienced users can also benefit from the deeper discussions on advanced topics like blending techniques and therapeutic applications. Additionally, these communities often host workshops, webinars, and meet-ups, providing opportunities for hands-on learning and net-working. Engaging with an essential oil community fosters a sense of belonging and can greatly enhance your understanding and appreciation of the vast world of essential oils.

21

Conclusion

In conclusion, our journey through the "Quick Guide to Essential Oils" has illuminated the multifaceted world of these aromatic extracts. From understanding their extraction and unique properties to exploring their versatile applications in aromatherapy, skincare, household cleaning, and natural remedies, we have uncovered the essence of what makes these oils a staple in natural wellness practices.

As we wrap up, remember that the journey with essential oils is one of continuous learning and discovery. Starting with a few essential oils, like lavender, peppermint, and lemon, can open doors to a universe of natural fragrances and benefits. Blending oils, experimenting with different uses, and joining communities further enrich this experience, offering endless possibilities for personal and household wellness.

Quality and safety remain paramount in this journey. Choosing high-quality, pure oils from reputable sources and adhering to safety guidelines ensures that the benefits of these natural wonders are enjoyed to their fullest. As you integrate these oils into your life, remember to do your research, and to consult health and wellness professionals for tailored advice as needed, especially for specific health concerns.

In essence, essential oils are nature's gift, offering a holistic approach to well-being. They invite us to connect with the natural world in a profound way, enhancing our daily lives with their therapeutic properties and delightful aromas. May this guide serve as your starting point in a journey that promises to be as enriching and enjoyable as the scents themselves. Embrace the natural elegance of essential oils and discover the myriad ways they can enhance your world.

If you found this book helpful, I would appreciate it if you would leave a favorable review for the book on Amazon. Thank you very much in advance.

Resources

Aromatherapist, J. L.-. C., & Aromatherapist, J. L.-. C. (2023, September 22). *What are the Most Popular Essential Oils? Nature's Aromatic Gems.* https://www.lovingessentialoils.com/blogs/aromatherapy-news/what-are-the-most-popular-essential-oils

Aromatherapy: Do essential oils really work? (2021, August 8). Johns Hopkins Medicine. https://www.hopkinsmedicine.org/health/wellness-and-prevention/aromatherapy-do-essential-oils-really-work

Banks, J. (2022, January 28). Roman Chamomile Essential Oil: 10 Uses and Benefits. *Essential Oil Tree.* https://www.essentialoiltree.com/roman-chamomile-essential-oil/

Bcps, R. P. P. B. B. (2023, May 5). *Eucalyptus: Everything you need to know.* Verywell Health. https://www.verywellhealth.com/eucalyptus-uses-benefits-side-effects-dosage-7483449

Capritto, A. (2020, November 4). The dangers of essential oils: Why natural isn't always safe. *CNET.* https://www.cnet.com/health/are-essential-oils-actually-safe/

Carter, E. (2023, November 17). *Top 10 best Essential oil brands in 2023.* Essential Oil Haven. https://www.essentialoilhaven.com/best-essential-oil-brands/

Carter, E., & Carter, E. (2021, October 31). *Top 10 lavender essential oil Benefits*. Essential Oil Haven. https://www.essentialoilhaven.com/top-10-lavender-essential-oil-benefits/

CCA, S. S. M. (2018, August 30). *A guide to essential oil safety.* Herbal Academy. https://theherbalacademy.com/a-guide-to-essential-oil-safety/

Cde, P. P. M. R. L. (2023, May 5). *9 Unexpected benefits of eucalyptus oil.* Healthline. https://www.healthline.com/health/9-ways-eucalyptus-oil-can-help

Cronkleton, E. (2019, March 8). *Aromatherapy Uses and benefits.* Healthline. https://www.healthline.com/health/what-is-aromatherapy

Deckard, A. (2016, May 31). *11 Proven rosemary essential oil Benefits.* Healthy Focus. https://healthyfocus.org/proven-benefits-rosemary-essential-oil/

Deckard, A. (2018, April 21). *16 Proven benefits of Eucalyptus essential Oil.* Healthy Focus. https://healthyfocus.org/eucalyptus-essential-oil/

Essential oil safety (And are essential oil diffusers safe?) - Dr. Axe. (2020, October 14). Dr. Axe. https://draxe.com/essential-oils/essential-oil-safety/

Eucalyptus oil benefits and uses - Dr. Axe. (2022, January 11). Dr. Axe. https://draxe.com/essential-oils/eucalyptus-oil-uses-benefits/

Exploring Aromatherapy | NAHA. (n.d.). https://naha.org/explore-aromatherapy/about-aromatherapy/what-is-aromatherapy//

Frankincense oil Benefits, uses and side effects - Dr. Axe. (2023, December 13). Dr. Axe. https://draxe.com/essential-oils/what-is-frankincense/

Lavender oil benefits and how to use it - Dr. Axe. (2023, January 31). Dr. Axe. https://draxe.com/essential-oils/lavender-oil-benefits/

Lemon essential oil Benefits, uses, side effects, DIY recipes - Dr. Axe. (2023, November 15). Dr. Axe. https://draxe.com/essential-oils/lemon-essential-oil-uses-benefits/

Living, Y. (2022, December 14). Our top essential oils to add to your collection. *Young Living Blog - US EN.* https://www.youngliving.com/blog/top-10-must-have-essential-oils/

Martin, G. (2021, October 1). *What are the 10 most popular essential oils?* Edens Garden. https://www.edensgarden.com/blogs/news/what-are-the-10-most-popular-essential-oils

mindbodygreen. (2023, April 18). *Benefits of lavender oil: 8 uses for this essential oil.* Mindbodygreen. https://www.mindbodygreen.com/articles/benefits-of-lavender

Nagdeve, M. (2020a, January 29). *13 Amazing benefits of Sandalwood Essential Oil.* Organic Facts. https://www.organicfacts.net/health-benefits/essential-oils/sandalwood-essential-oil.html

Nagdeve, M. (2020b, January 29). *31 Surprising peppermint oil Benefits & Uses.* Organic Facts. https://www.organicfacts.net/health-benefits/essential-oils/health-benefits-of-peppermint-oil.html

Nagdeve, M. (2021, July 22). *11 Surprising benefits of Chamomile essential oil.* Organic Facts. https://www.organicfacts.net/health-benefits/esse ntial-oils/camomile-essential-oil.html

Nagdeve, M., & Nagdeve, M. (2020, October 8). *10 Health benefits of Frankincense essential oil.* Organic Facts. https://www.organicfacts.net/ health-benefits/essential-oils/health-benefits-of-frankincense-esse ntial-oil.html

Peppermint oil uses, benefits, side effects and more - Dr. Axe. (2023, December 8). Dr. Axe. https://draxe.com/essential-oils/peppermint-oil-uses-benefits/

Professional, C. C. M. (n.d.). *Aromatherapy.* Cleveland Clinic. https://my. clevelandclinic.org/health/treatments/aromatherapy

Pugle, M. (2019, April 26). *Are essential oils safe? 13 things to know Before use.* Healthline. https://www.healthline.com/health/are-essential-oil s-safe

Rd, M. M. M. (2023, March 17). *14 Benefits and Uses of rosemary essential oil.* Healthline. https://www.healthline.com/nutrition/rosemary-oil-benefits

Rosemary Benefits, uses, side effects, interactions and more - Dr. Axe. (2021, September 6). Dr. Axe. https://draxe.com/nutrition/rosemary-benefit s/

Sandalwood essential oil Benefits and uses - Dr. Axe. (2023, September 20). Dr. Axe. https://draxe.com/essential-oils/sandalwood-essential-oil/

Schaefer, A. (2021, August 2). *The health potential of sandalwood.*

Healthline. https://www.healthline.com/health/what-is-sandalwood

Seladi-Schulman, J., PhD. (2019, August 14). *The 8 proven benefits of chamomile oil and how to use it.* Healthline. https://www.healthline.com/health/chamomile-oil

Seladi-Schulman, J., PhD. (2023, April 4). *Peppermint oil uses and benefits.* Healthline. https://www.healthline.com/health/benefits-of-peppermint-oil

Seward, M. (2016, November 10). *The top 10 benefits of lemon essential oil.* Healthy Focus. https://healthyfocus.org/top-10-benefits-of-lemon-essential-oil/

Seward, M. (2018, November 27). *11 Proven Ylang ylang essential oil Benefits.* Healthy Focus. https://healthyfocus.org/ylang-ylang-essential-oil-benefits/

Seward, M. (2019, May 26). *21 proven tea tree essential oil benefits.* Healthy Focus. https://healthyfocus.org/tea-tree-essential-oil-benefits/

Seward, M. (2023, September 2). *11 Proven frankincense essential oil Benefits.* Healthy Focus. https://healthyfocus.org/frankincense-essential-oil-benefits/

TEA TREE OIL: Overview, uses, side effects, precautions, interactions, dosing and reviews. (n.d.). https://www.webmd.com/vitamins/ai/ingredientmono-113/tea-tree-oil

The Healthline Editorial Team. (2023, February 6). *14 everyday uses for tea tree oil.* Healthline. https://www.healthline.com/nutrition/tea-tree-oil

Watson, K. (2023, May 31). *What you need to know about lemon Essential oil*. Healthline. https://www.healthline.com/health/lemon-essential-oil

WebMD Editorial Contributors. (2020, December 14). *Health benefits of frankincense essential oil*. WebMD. https://www.webmd.com/diet/health-benefits-frankincense-essential-oil

Whelan, C. (2023, July 13). *About Ylang Ylang Essential Oil*. Healthline. https://www.healthline.com/health/ylang-ylang

Ylang Ylang Benefits, uses, recipes and side effects - Dr. Axe. (2019, November 7). Dr. Axe. https://draxe.com/essential-oils/ylang-ylang/

www.ingramcontent.com/pod-product-compliance
Lightning Source LLC
Chambersburg PA
CBHW040258240726
48664CB00006B/1285